for the children in my class and
around the world who give us all
joy and hope

dedicated to
Russell and Rose who fill our
home with music, art, and love

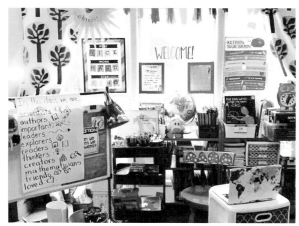

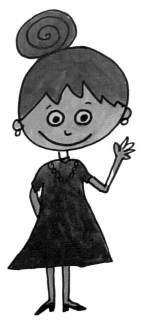

School may look different this year.

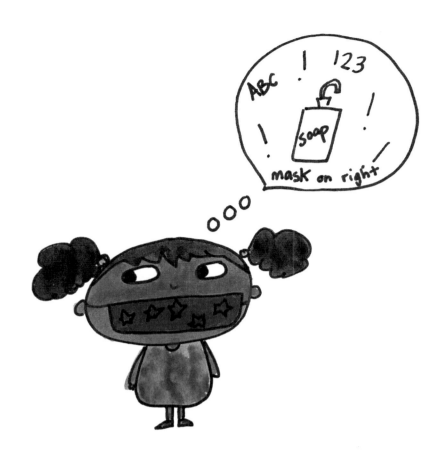

There will be many
things to remember.
Here are a few do's
and don'ts to guide you
along your way.

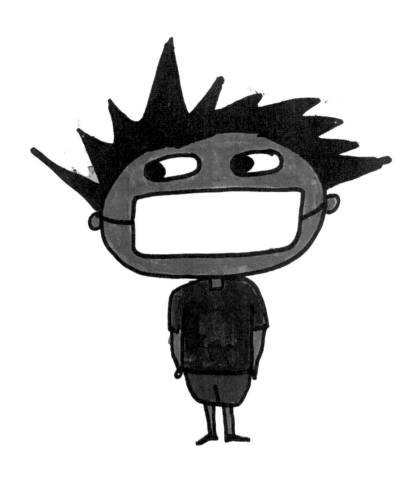

Do wear a mask
on your face.

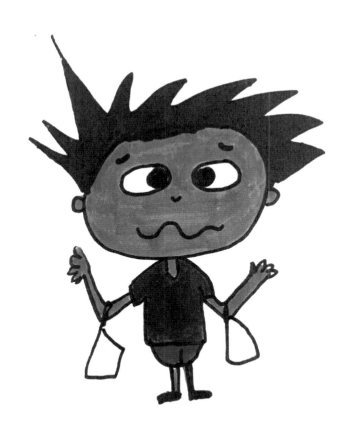

Don't wear a mask
on your elbows.

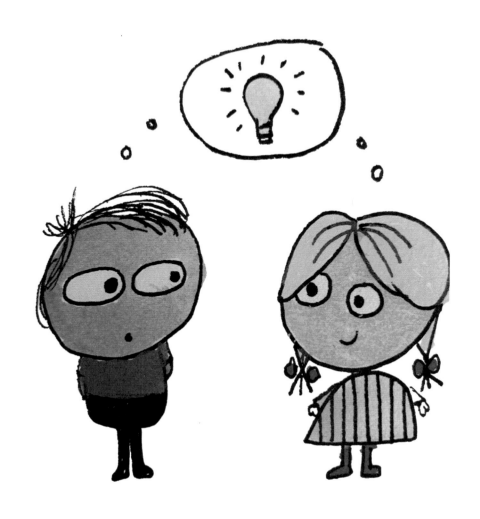

Do share ideas.

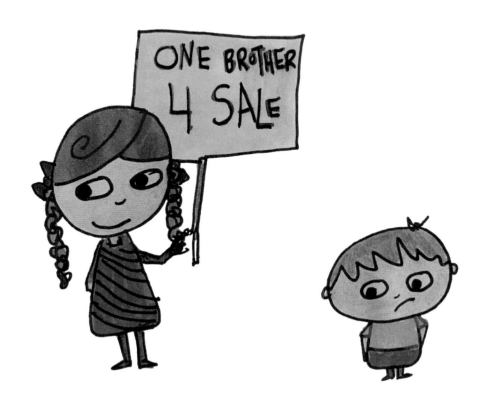

Don't share your brother.

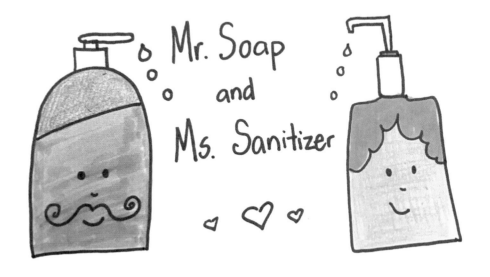

Do wash your hands
with soap and sanitizer.

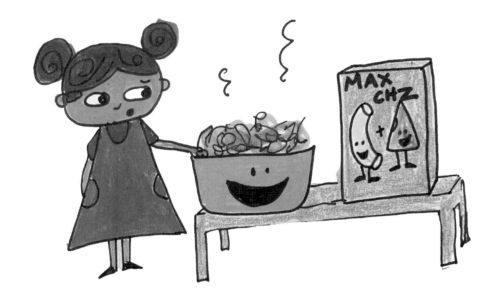

Don't wash your hands
with macaroni and
cheese.

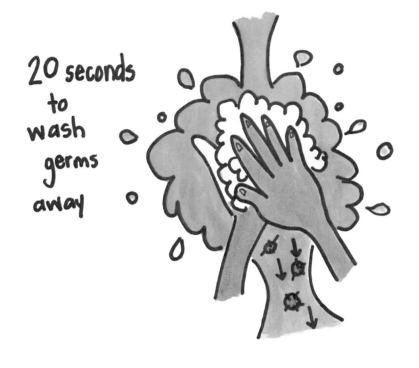

20 seconds
to
wash
germs
away

Do wash your hands
for 20 seconds.

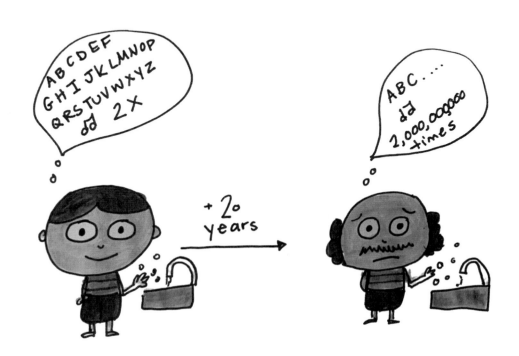

Don't wash your hands
for 20 years.

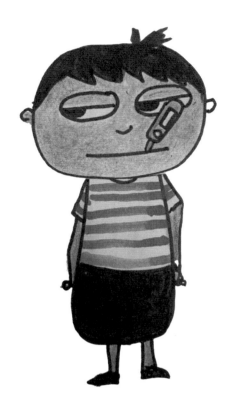

Do stay home when you don't feel well.

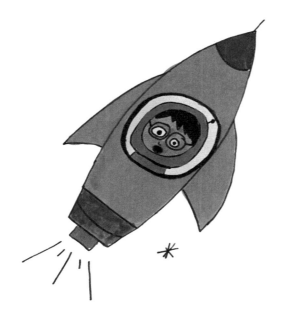

Don't fly to outer space
when you don't feel well.

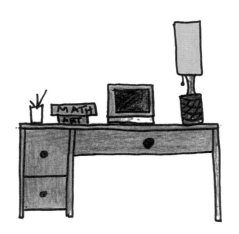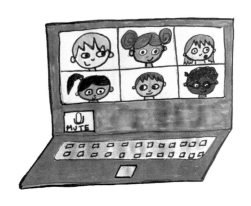

Do work hard in class and
at home.

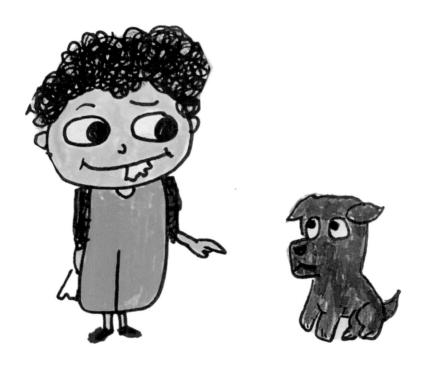

Don't eat your homework.

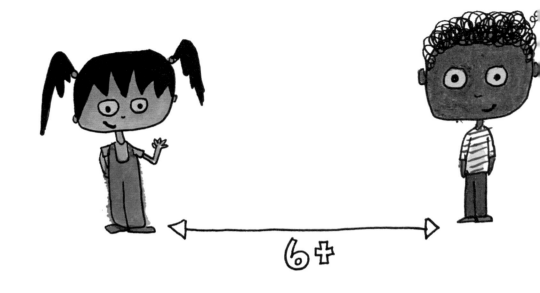

feet

Do stay safely apart.

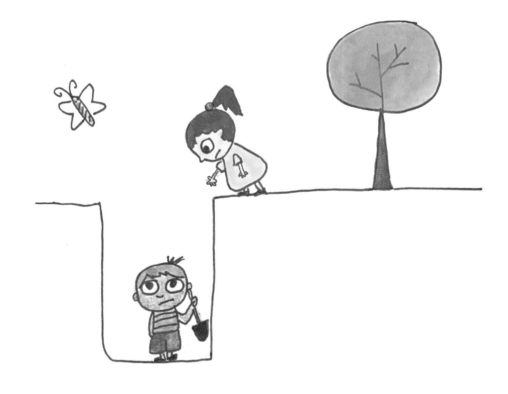

Don't do it by digging a
hole under the playground

.

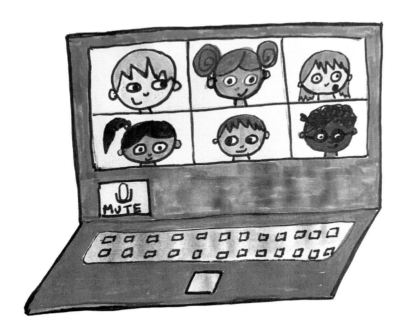

Do join in on class
meetings.

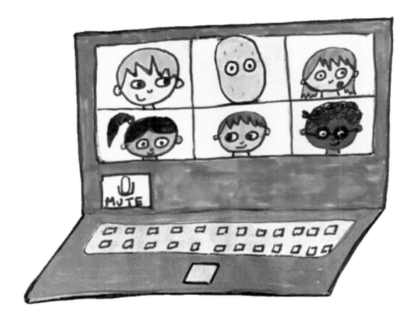

Don't turn your
picture into a
potato.

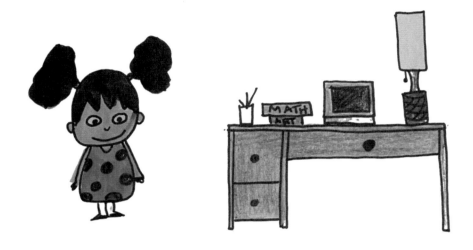

Do find a good place
to learn.

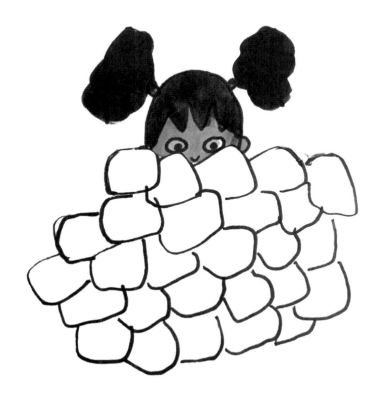

Don't make it out of
marshmallows.

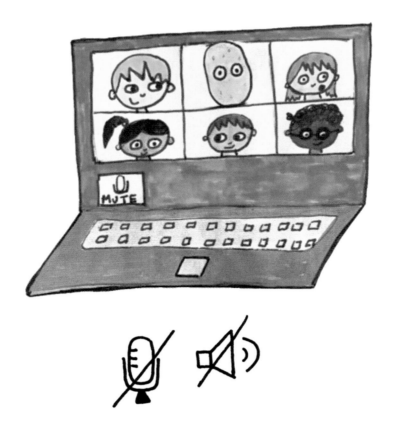

Do mute yourself
sometimes.

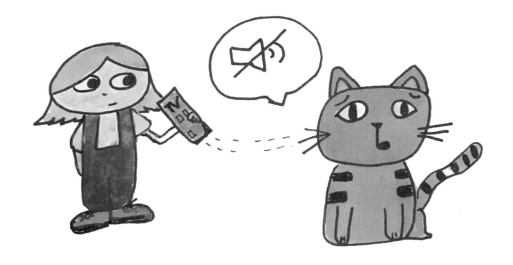

Don't mute your cat.

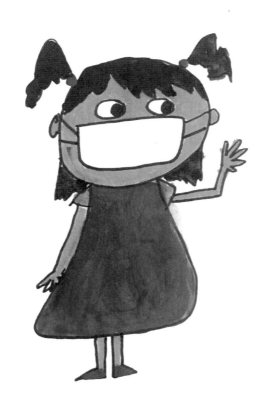

Do keep your hands
off your face.

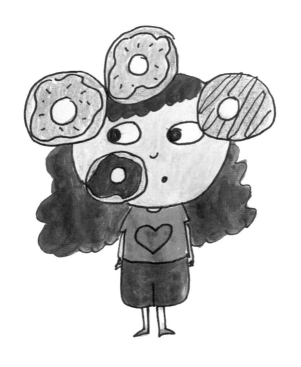

Don't put donuts on
your face.

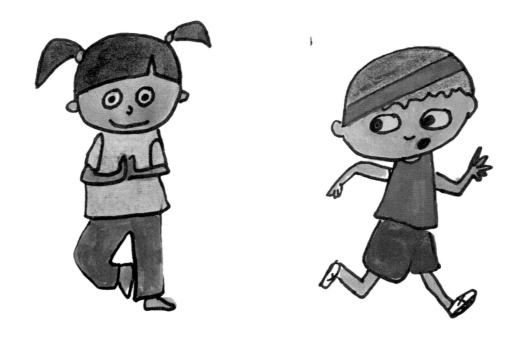

Do exercise to stay
healthy.

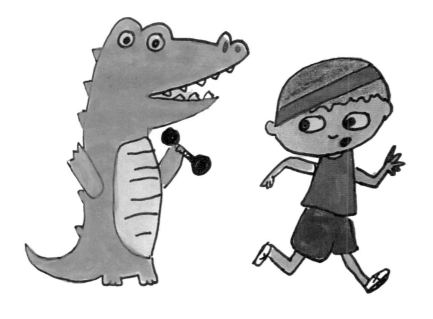

Don't exercise with an
alligator.

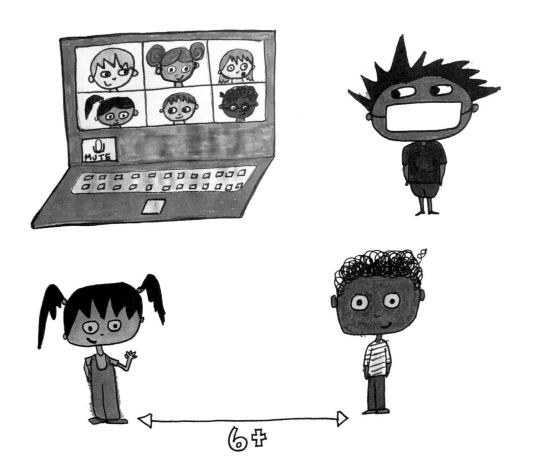

Even though some
things are different....

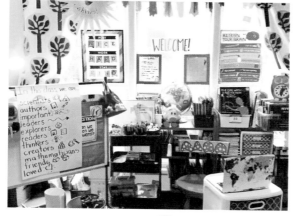

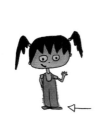 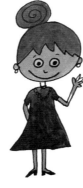 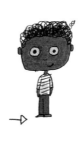

Others remain the same. We keep laughing, learning, and loving each other.

Made in the USA
Monee, IL
20 July 2020